THE ABCs

Of

MENOPAUSE

GILLIANNE FULLER

Copyright © 2022 by Gillianne Fuller

All rights reserved. No part of this book may be reproduced or used in any manner without written permission of the copyright owner except for the use of quotations in a book review.

CONTENTS

Introduction v

Chapter 1: Menopause 9

Chapter 2: The Symptoms 16

Chapter 3: The Solutions 26

Summary 49

References 50

INTRODUCTION

By 2025, there will be an estimated 1 billion women in the world experiencing menopause, and yet there is such a stigma surrounding menopause that it is rarely spoken about. Women rarely talk about their symptoms or are just unsure as to what is happening to them. Some women believe that what they are experiencing is normal, and they will just have to live with these changes for the rest of their lives. Despite the increasing information in recent years, there is still so much more to learn. There is a lack of education and a lack of resources, women are left in the dark. One day, we are suddenly hit by these symptoms that we believe are normal. We begin to believe that we have to live with them for the rest of our lives. Our GP doesn't understand what we are going through. They want to prescribe antidepressants and send us off to any specialists they can think of.

A lot of women feel that it is the end of life as they knew it. Marriages are failing, and according to a survey, over 60 percent of divorces are initiated by women in their perimenopausal/menopausal years. Women are leaving their careers of decades, or not accepting promotions. Studies show that 99% of women felt that menopause harmed their careers. More than 50% of the women surveyed took some time off due to menopausal symptoms. We have little or no support in the workplace and fear disclosing our menopausal status because we fear the stigma that comes with menopause.

We are too ashamed to discuss our menopause symptoms with our husbands, girlfriends, or even our doctors. Let's face it, a lot of mothers did not even talk about menopause, they suffered in silence so a lot of us are not even sure what we are experiencing. A lot of women never seek help. My mother told me recently that she has been having menopausal symptoms for over 35 years. I am sure there are millions of women just like her. It is time for a change, and it is time to talk about it more and educate ourselves more so we can begin to remove the stigma surrounding it. With the right information, foods, nutrition, exercise, and programs created specifically for you; this can be another great chapter of your life.

Firstly, did you even know there were different stages of menopause? Perimenopause, Menopause, and Post-menopause; I sure did not. At 53 years old, I knew nothing about menopause. It hit me like a ton of bricks one day. I had to get online quickly and research that fire that had just started in my head and was slowly traveling to my lower body. I got scared and nervous, and I thought "OMG, what the hell is happening to me, is this some type of illness." Google told me that it may be hot flashes, and I thought thanked God for Google.

I realized then that even though most of my women friends were around the same age as I was, I had never heard any of them mention menopause or any of the symptoms related to menopause. I decided then that it was time to get the conversation started. We do not want the next generation to be as lost as we are. We want to ensure that our daughters know that the earlier they start living a healthier lifestyle, eating the right foods, getting enough sleep, exercising, and taking the right vitamins and supplements, the easier this time of life will be.

And so began my journey to get as many people to talk about menopause as possible. I started a Clubhouse Club called **Women over 50, Let's Talk Menopause and Life after 50.** I started a non-profit organization called Menopause Matter; www.menopausematter.org and I decide to write a short simple-to-read guide to understand the menopausal journey. Hope it will help!

CHAPTER 1

MENOPAUSE

Menopause is the second phase in the cycle and begins when a woman has not had a menstrual period for one full year/12 consecutive months. Menopause is not an illness, it is a natural biological process that cannot be treated; however, the symptoms associated with it can be treated.

Studies show that menopause symptoms may last an average of 4-5 years following a person's last period and a total of 7.4 years in total. Menopause, however, is just one day, it is the day your period officially ends, and the day after begins the third cycle, post-menopause.

Menopause should be permanent, and you should not see the return of your menstrual period. If you do, see your physician immediately.

Women will spend about 1/3 of their lives in a menopausal state, so we need to make sure we maintain the quality of life we had before. A lot of our menopausal symptoms can be helped with diet, exercise, and the right lifestyle.

Menopause usually happens in your 40s or 50s, but it can also happen as early as in your 30s and on occasion even in your 20s. About 1 in every 1000 women will reach menopause before the age of 30. This is called premature menopause. Medical treatments such as chemotherapy or some surgeries like removal of the ovaries can induce early menopause. Other causes may include autoimmune conditions such as Crohn's disease, chromosome defects such as Tuner's syndrome, or genetic factors; most likely if your mother had non-medically induced early menopause, you will as well.

There are also cases where a woman's ovaries just randomly stop producing eggs, this is called POI or Premature Ovarian Insufficiency. These women with premature menopause will usually have a long perimenopausal life. The symptoms of premature menopause are the same as natural menopause.

A longer perimenopausal life comes with more health risks such as early-onset osteoporosis, heart disease, and an increased risk of developing type 2 diabetes.

There is no treatment to make your ovaries start working again, but studies show that one in every ten women that have POI will get pregnant.

Studies also show that women who have never been pregnant have more of a chance of having menopause before 40.

Perimenopause

Perimenopause is the first stage in the cycle and can begin as early as 8 to 10 years before menopause.

Perimenopause can start as early as in your 30s but as late as in your 50s. It is the period leading up to menopause. In perimenopause, the ovaries gradually begin to make less estrogen, the main female hormone in the body, and your menstrual period begins to get erratic, it may lengthen or shorten. You may skip some periods, or the flow may get heavier. Perimenopause varies from one woman to the next. On average, it last three to four years but can be as short as a few years or as long as a decade. Some women will have a slew of symptoms while some women will have none.

Progesterone hormones are chemical messengers produced by the ovaries, adrenals, and placenta. Its main role concerns menstruation and pregnancy but has other functions such as protecting the lining of your womb, acting as a sedative for sleep, regulating mood, and helping with anxiety. It will also help with skin dryness, thinning, and wrinkling of the skin. Helps to fight weight gain and prevent the loss of bone density. Helps regulate blood pressure and supports cognition. During perimenopause, your progesterone production begins to fluctuate. Low progesterone will affect all these functions during perimenopause.

Estrogen is the main group of hormones that plays a role in female sexual and reproductive development. The estrogen hormone in a woman is primarily produced by the woman's ovaries. Your natural estrogen production will change over time. During your childbearing years and puberty, you produce a lot of estrogens, but as menopause approaches, your estrogen production begins to decline.

When your estrogen level drops significantly, it may trigger some symptoms of perimenopause. One of the first signs of perimenopause is an unpredictable menstrual cycle. Women can go from a very predictable cycle to an erratic cycle.

Some symptoms are:

- Heavy bleeding—25% of women will experience heavy bleeding.
- Hot flashes—83% of women will experience hot flashes.
- Vaginal dryness—more than 50% of women between 51 and 60 will experience vaginal dryness.
- Brain fog—92% will experience forgetfulness.
- Insomnia—94% of women will have difficulty sleeping.
- Anger/mood swings—87% of females will experience mood swings and irritability.
- Depression—28% of women in perimenopause and 59% of women will have a history of depression
- Night sweats—86% will have night sweats.
- Incontinence—more than 50% of menopausal women will have incontinence.
- Loss of bone—1 in 10 women over the age of 60 will experience bone loss.
- Headaches—more than 25% of women will experience migraine headaches.

And more...

There are said to be more than 100 possible symptoms of perimenopause, and while I will not be going into details about them all, these are also a few of the lesser common symptoms:

- Body odour may change
- Bloating
- Breast tenderness
- Dizziness
- Electric shock sensation/pins and needles sensation
- Joint pains
- Oral problems
- Allergies
- Hair loss
- Hair dryness and fizziness
- Weight gain
- Panic attacks
- Fatigue
- Lower libido
- Dizzy spells
- Itchy skin
- Brittle nails
- Memory lapse
- Acid reflux
- Restless legs

- Heart palpitations
- Sensitive teeth
- Acne
- Dry eyes
- Breathlessness
- Sore breast
- Vertigo
- Digestive issues
- Tense muscles
- Facial hair
- Bad breath
- Weight loss
- Dry mouth
- Bleeding gums

Post-menopause

If you have gone without any menstrual cycle for one year, that is 12 consecutive months, you are in menopause. The next day, you begin post-menopause. Post-menopause can last 4 to 5 years after menopause, but every woman is different.

Post-menopause begins after menopause. In post-menopause, you can no longer become pregnant, no more menstrual cycles, and hormone levels remain low. In post-menopause, you can still experience the symptoms faced during perimenopause. Your perimenopausal symptoms may begin to subside at this time but may also continue for years.

Post-menopausal women are at a greater risk of heart disease, osteoporosis, and bone loss. Estrogen helps protect against heart disease, heart attacks, and strokes. Women in post-menopause tend to be more inanimate or immobile; therefore, there is more of a risk of high blood pressure and high cholesterol which can lead to cardiovascular diseases.

More women suffer from fractured hips and problems related to bone density after menopause. Women can lose up to 25% of their bone density, this increases the risk of bone fractures. Your hips, wrist, and spine are the most commonly affected areas. Women should make sure they take a bone density test once every two years to check for early signs of osteoporosis and take calcium daily.

During your post-menopausal years, you should have regular mammograms, breast exams, pap smears, and pelvic exams.

CHAPTER 2

THE SYMPTOMS

Heavy bleeding

It is quite common to have heavy bleeding and even blood clots during perimenopause, these heavy periods are called menorrhagia. The hormonal ups and downs of perimenopause can cause any bleeding pattern you can think of. You may have shorter cycles or more frequent cycles. One period may be just ending, and before you know it, another one starts. You may miss a period only for it to return twice as heavy as normal. Every woman is different and will have different experiences.

In a study of more than 1300 perimenopausal women, over 91% have experienced at least one occurrence of heavy bleeding lasting 3 or more days. 25% reported heavy bleeding lasting 10 or more days during six months.

When there is an imbalance in your hormone levels—your estrogen levels are high, and your progesterone levels are low—your uterine lining builds resulting in heavy bleeding during your periods. A missed period can also cause the uterine lining to build leading to heavy bleeding.

It's considered heavy bleeding when you soak through a pad an hour for several hours. Or when you need to use both a pad and a tampon at the same time for double protection. When you bleed for more than a week or when you have to interrupt your sleep to change your pad.

Although heavy bleeding during perimenopause is normal, if your heavy bleeding persists, see your doctor as there can be other causes, and it can lead to you becoming anemic from blood loss. If you experience clots larger than a quarter, and you have **bleeding after menopause,** bleeding that lasts more than two weeks—accompanied by dizziness, breathlessness, or fatigue—see your doctor immediately.

Hot flashes

Hot flushes are one of the most common symptoms of perimenopause. They come on quickly and can last from one to five minutes. Some women can experience up the 30 hot flashes per day. They range in severity from just feeling warm and flushed to feeling like a fire has started inside your body. Some women will also have an aura or warning that a hot flash is about to occur. A severe hot flash can leave you sweating and give you chills. I have even experienced anxiety just before a hot flash. Hot flashes are an intense feeling of heat coming from your body, usually your face, neck, and chest. Leaving you flushed, and in some cases, even drenched in perspiration. Over 40% of women in their 40s start to experience hot flashes. The severity depends on the individual. 80% will stop having it after 5years while others will experience hot flashes for 10-15 years.

Some women will have mild hot flashes while other women are unable to function normally, they are unable to keep schedules or hold meetings because of the severity of their hot flashes. The cause of hot flashes is not known exactly but is believed to have been caused by "the brain's thermoregulatory center which controls heat production and loss and is influenced by hormones" according to John Hopkins Medicine.

According to The Mayo Clinic, women who smoke, women who are obese, and black women report more frequency of hot flashes while Asian women report having the least number of hot flashes. Their research also suggests that women who have hot flashes have an increased risk of heart disease and greater bone loss.

Vaginal Dryness

As the estrogen level lowers, the vagina's tissues begin to get thinner, less elastic, and drier. This leads to vaginal dryness, itching, burning, and you may need to urinate more or have urinary tract infections more often. This can also cause pain during intercourse, sports, and other physical activity. 58% of women will experience vaginal dryness after menopause. Note, that vaginal dryness can happen at any age due to some different causes such as breastfeeding, cigarette smoking, depression, childbirth, chemotherapy, removal of the ovaries, and excessive stress. Vaginal dryness may cause burning, loss of interest in sex, pain during intercourse, light bleeding following intercourse, UTI (urinary tract infection), and itching/stinging. In some cases, vaginal dryness may also cause pain when you sit, stand, or urinate. You may also experience a shorter and tighter vaginal canal and a dry dark red colored vagina lining.

Vaginal dryness is rarely serious, and some treatments can treat it and even ways to try to prevent it; however, it can have life-changing effects on women. Many women are so confused and embarrassed by their symptoms that they refuse to talk about them even to their partners. This can put a strain on their relationship especially if they are unwilling to tell their partner why they are not interested in sex. Recognizing that your vaginal dryness is common is the first step to helping yourself.

Brain Fog

Forgetfulness, difficulty in concentrating, and thinking clearly. Your memory does not feel sharp, and you have trouble focusing. Between the age of 45 and 55, a women's performance on certain memory tasks dips as the level of estrogen drops. Studies show that women with low levels of estrogen do badly in a memory test. Studies also show that women in their first year of their last menstrual period had the lowest score on the test for verbal learning, motor function, attention, and working memory tasks. Memory issues during your stages of menopause are normal, over 60% of women will experience these issues.

Although menopause brain fog will not last forever, it can stick around for years. Women may not feel as focused for a few years. Studies show that women have trouble concentrating, trouble finding the right words, and mention feeling foggy. Remember, estrogen is the "master regulator" of our brain. Our brain has a lot of estrogen receptors so when our estrogen levels are low, it has a profound impact on the functions of our brain.

Insomnia

People with insomnia may take up to 30 minutes to fall asleep. Get less than 6 hours of sleep on three or more nights per week. They will not feel rested after sleeping. They will wake too early and will feel sleepy and tired throughout the day.

Studies have shown that up 60% of women going through menopause will experience these sleep issues.

- Difficulty falling asleep.
- Difficulty staying asleep.
- Early morning awakening.
- Less total sleep time.
- Fatigue during the day.
- Non-restorative sleep.

The decline of estrogen can cause hot flashes, night sweats, depression, and anxiety which could lead to disruptive sleep. Having bladder issues is another result of estrogen decline, and the frequent need to pass urine at night is also another reason for sleep disturbances. Melatonin is a vital hormone necessary for sleep, and with age, its production decreases which may also cause sleep disturbances. Progesterone is a sleep-producing hormone, so the decline in progesterone will also affect your ability to fall asleep and stay asleep.

Anger

Mood swings and anger are very real symptoms of perimenopause. The stress of lack of sleep, hot flashes, and everything else going on combined with low hormone levels can cause anxiety, stress, anger, and moods that are unstable. Estrogen controls the production of serotonin in your brain, so low estrogen will also mean low serotonin. Serotonin is the chemical that helps to regulate your mood.

Our periods are unpredictable, no one is talking about their symptoms, so we feel alone, sleep is rare, bladder control may be a problem, sex may hurt or be non-existent, and we may be losing our hair, or it's dry and brittle. We may be gaining weight around your midsection. We may feel depressed. These things will all contribute to us sometimes feeling angry.

Depression

Depression is another common symptom of perimenopause. It is known that during drops in estrogen levels such as around the time of childbirth, women can experience depression. Remember, estrogen is responsible for starting the menstruation cycle, development in females, regulating sex drive, controlling weight gain and metabolism, managing the growth of the uterine lining, and more. When estrogen production starts to decline, all these functions are disrupted, and depression can be a result.

Some women may feel mildly irritated or sad while other women will be severely depressed and unable to function in their normal daily lives. Major depression is associated with a chemical imbalance in the brain, and the change in our hormone levels during perimenopause may contribute to that imbalance. According to NAMS, if you experience any of the following symptoms all day every day for more than two weeks, then you are believed to be depressed and should seek medical help:

- Feeling hopeless
- Loss of energy; tired
- Moving or talking more slowly
- Feeling helpless, unworthy, and guilty
- Persistently sad or anxious
- Feeling worthless
- Loss of appetite and weight change
- Headaches, aches, pains, and digestive issues with no medical cause
- Difficulty making decisions, concentrating and remembering
- Loss of interest or pleasure in things that you would normally love
- Thoughts of death or suicide or suicide attempts

Mood swings

According to a NAMS Study, up to 23% of women in menopause has mood swings. One minute you are happy, the next you are sad. Women suffer from anxiety, irritability, crying episodes, feeling weepy, and you may not feel as confident as before.

Menopausal women tend to find themselves irritated easily; things that may not have bothered them previously may now become more annoying. We worry more, may have panic attacks, and experience more tension and nervousness. You may find yourself crying over something that wouldn't have mattered previous to menopause.

A reduced level of estrogen causes mood swings. The mood swings can be mild but can also lead up to aggression.

Night Sweats

Night sweats are not hot flashes. Night sweats are a period of heavy sweating that occurs at night due to hot flashes. Night sweats will jolt you from your sleep and even leave the sheets so wet that you will have to change the sheets and nightclothes. Sweating is your body trying to get rid of excess heat. So, the night sweats are a result of the buildup of heat from the hot flashes.

Some women will only experience night sweats for a few years while others will experience night sweats for even a decade, every woman will experience perimenopause differently.

Incontinence

Incontinence is losing the ability to control your bladder. One of the major reasons that the bladder leaks is a weakened pelvic muscle, this is called pelvic relaxation. As the body produces less and less estrogen, it causes a thinning of the urethra, and your pelvic muscles begin to weaken. Estrogen helps to keep the connective tissues of the pelvis and the urinary tract healthy, so without enough estrogen, the support to the bladder and urethra weakens.

Stress incontinence is when your bladder leaks when you cough, sneeze, or exercise.

Urge incontinence can cause a sudden intense need to urinate—needing to urinate throughout the night. Urge incontinence may be caused by an infection.

Overflow incontinence is when your bladder does not empty fully so you have a constant dripping of urine.

Functional incontinence is when a physical or mental impairment prevents you from getting to the bathroom on time.

Mixed incontinence is when you experience more than one type of incontinence.

Overactive bladder is caused by an irritation in the bladder which causes urgency and frequency.

Bone Loss

There are an estimated 10 million Americans with osteoporosis, and of those 10 million, 80% are women. Women tend to have smaller bones than men so more prone to osteoporosis. Estrogen also protects our bones so when a woman reaches menopause, and her estrogen levels decrease sharply, there is a greater risk of bone loss.

Studies show that one in two women over the age of 50 will break a bone because of osteoporosis. Also, Caucasian women may be more prone to osteoporosis.

More than 50% of Caucasian women over 50 years of age are estimated to have low bone mass. 5% of African American women are estimated to have osteoporosis, and 35% are estimated to have low bone mass. Also, because African American women tend to stay out of the sun, they have low vitamin D levels, and that can make it hard for the body to absorb calcium.

For some women, their bone loss can be rapid. The greater your bone density is before reaching menopause will determine your risk of getting osteoporosis after menopause. Also, some women will lose bone density rapidly. A woman can lose up to 20% of her bone density during the first five to seven years following menopause.

CHAPTER 3

THE SOLUTIONS

Heavy Bleeding

Heavy bleeding also known as menorrhagia or hypermenorrhea is common among women transitioning into menopause. A healthy lifestyle, sleep management, and balanced hormones can help with your heavy bleeding. Manage your stress level so you do not have a further hormone imbalance. Keep a journal so you have better knowledge and control over your blood flow.

Eat more foods rich in iron or ask your doctor about iron supplements. Some foods rich in iron are shellfish, beef, spinach, beans, dark leafy vegetables, peas, chicken, veal, perch, salmon, liver, raisins, apricots, soybeans, iron-fortified loaves of bread, and cereals. Also eating foods rich in vitamin C will help your body's ability to absorb iron. Some foods rich in vitamin C are citrus fruits, melons, strawberries, chili peppers, mangoes, and sweet peppers.

You can always speak to your doctor about other methods that may help to reduce your heavy bleeding such as a low dose birth control pill. HRT is an option some women choose; it will not only help with your heavy bleeding but also with your other perimenopausal symptoms as well. You and your doctor or medical professional can work together to find a product that works for you. Remember, every woman is different so what works for your sister may not work for you.

Try Reiki, homeopathic remedies, and deep-tissue massages all of which may help with the pain and other symptoms associated with heavy bleeding. For the pains associated with heavy bleeding, try a heating pad, the warmth will help relax the muscles involved. Stay hydrated, heavy periods also cause the body to lose a lot of water.

Hot Flashes

Using nature's estrogen which is found in soy products may help with your hot flashes. Foods such as tofu, flax seeds, and edamame. Studies have shown that black cohosh may be helpful for short periods. Exercising daily will help—doing yoga, dancing, and walking. Practicing deep breathing and slow abdominal breathing.

Yoga, restorative, and supportive poses may improve your symptoms. Yoga can also help muscle loss and degenerating joints. The poses of restorative yoga will relax the body and help to relax the nervous system.

Exercise is always a good idea. Physical activity will cause the brain to release neurotransmitters like serotonin and dopamine which also affects things like mood and mental sharpness. Studies also show that exercise changes the blood flow to the skin and brain and could influence how the brain regulates temperature. Exercise will help you to lose that perimenopausal weight and strengthen your bones.

Flaxseed is said to help with not only your hot flashes but to reduce the risk of osteoporosis—weakening of the bones. **Flaxseeds are high in phytoestrogens** that will help to regulate hot flashes and are said to improve the cardiovascular health of women by reducing blood pressure and preventing the hardening of the arteries.

Tofu, soybeans, soymilk, and edamame contain phytoestrogens which mimic biological estrogen and may help control hormone levels which may help reduce your hot flashes.

Sage contains flavonoids that may reduce the symptoms of hot flashes and promotes overall health.

Vitamin D is particularly important during perimenopause. Low vitamin D has been linked to osteoporosis and depression. Vitamin D functions more like a hormone than a vitamin and is not found in a lot of foods so we get our vitamin D from the sun or supplements. It is one of the most important vitamins for menopausal women. Vitamin D does so much for the woman's body, every woman over the age of 40 should ensure that she gets enough. Vitamin D will help you with your hot flashes but also with high blood pressure, heart disease, diabetes, and more. Studies suggest that you should get between 800 and 1000 IU of D3 per day. If you have fairer skin, you need 10-15mins in the sun and that could produce as much as 5000 IU. For darker skin, as much as six times longer depending on your skin pigmentation.

Vitamin B, B5, B2, B12, B6, and B3 helps to reduce the severity of hot flashes by regulating your hormones. Eat foods such as whole-grain loaves of bread and cereals. Avocados, nuts, eggs, bananas, sunflower seeds, green leafy veggies, nuts, and beans.

Red Clover contains isoflavone which helps in alleviating the symptoms of estrogen loss. It will help to control your hot flashes as well as other symptoms of menopause like bone loss, disturbed sleep, joint inflammation, osteoporosis, and heart disease.

Diet and nutrition are not only important for your hot flashes but your overall health. Bad dietary habits could affect your health and leaves a risk of developing certain diseases. Nutrition plays a role in balancing your hormones during perimenopause. A diet with whole foods, nutrient-rich foods, and foods with antioxidants, rich in color, berries, beans, and dark leafy greens should all help to lessen your symptoms.

Stay cool, use fans, and wear loose clothing, clothes made with natural fibers. Stay away from stress. Stress causes the release of a substance called epinephrine which increases the body temperature and causes sweating. Avoid caffeine, alcohol, and spicy foods. Try to quit smoking if you smoke. Stay hydrated, take cold showers, and running your face or wrist under cold water will quickly reduce the body temperature.

Keep a journal, identify your trigger points, and try to avoid them. Knowing which specific factors trigger your hot flashes will help you to better manage them.

Some women suffer severe hot flashes and may seek to have HRT—Hormone Replace Therapy. This will also help with other symptoms that you may face. You must speak to your doctor or medical professional before trying any treatments.

Vaginal Dryness

Some over-the-counter treatments may help with your vaginal dryness. Try using a water-based lubricant during intercourse. Water-based is better than oil-based because oil-based may irritate.

Try a lot of foreplay before intercourse to stimulate blood flow which will help to stimulate moisture. Also, having regular sex increases the blood flow to the genitals which keeps them healthy.

There are topical estrogen creams that can be applied directly to the vagina area to relieve your symptoms. There are vaginal estrogen rings that are inserted into the vagina and release low amounts of estrogen into the tissue. Vaginal estrogen tablet inserts where you use an applicator and place a tablet directly into the vagina.

Vaginal moisturizers are used about 2/3 times a wk. They last for up to 3 days.

A diet rich in fatty acids may help with your vaginal dryness. Raw pumpkin seeds, sesame seeds, sunflower seeds, salmon, mackerel, and tuna are high in fatty acids.

Avoid using too many perfumed soaps and powders etc. They can irritate the vagina and cause further dryness.

Quit smoking, it decreases estrogen levels.

Regular exercise aids in hormone balance.

Keep hydrated to maintain moisture levels in your body.

Try natural lubricants such as coconut oil, peanut oil, olive oil, and aloe vera. Note that natural oils are not recommended for use with latex condoms, they damage the latex and can lead to condom breakage.

Try essential oils such as jasmine, clary sage, lemon, fennel, rosemary, sweet orange, coriander, and carrot seeds. For example, lemon essential oil can heal and restore the dermal layer of the skin and is also an anti-inflammatory. Rosemary essential oil can stimulate the adrenal cortex which is the second source of estrogen in the body and becomes even more important during menopause.

Oral estrogen, HRT is also an option, see your medical provider.

Keep a journal and make a list of your questions. If there are things you do not understand ask questions. Do not be afraid to talk about it, millions of women are experiencing the same issues, and you are not alone.

Wear more cotton underwear and less synthetic ones, less risk of infections, and more comfortable.

Stop douching, the vaginal is a self-cleaning oven!

As always, your health care provider is the best source of information when it comes to medical issues

Brain Fog

Lifestyle changes may help with your brain fog.

Eat a well-balanced diet rich in whole foods and healthy fats. Not all fats are bad, the body needs some fats for energy to absorb vitamins and for heart and brain health. Healthy fats will help you to fight fatigue and help with your mental health so understanding the differences between good fats and bad fats is essential. Foods such as fish, nuts, beans, olive oil, vegetables, and fruits. Diets that include omega 3 fatty acids and unsaturated fats such as avocado, flaxseed, tofu, herring, sardines, almonds, hazelnuts, pumpkin seeds, sesame seeds, peanut, and soybeans.

Vitamin B6 and Vitamin B12 support cognitive function—the ability to think, reason, and remember—so getting enough of these vitamins is essential and may lower the risk of dementia developing over time. Vitamin B plays a role in the creation and activation of the estrogen in your body and is an especially important vitamin to consider during menopause.

If you are not sleeping well, your brain will not regenerate itself properly and that will affect the way your brain functions, so getting enough sleep is essential to good brain health. Get at least 7 hours of sleep per night. That 1 am to 4 am sleep is particularly important to your body's recovery.

Alleviate your stress. Use positive thinking.

Exercise

Spend less time at your computer and on your phone.

Balancing your hormones will help with the symptoms of menopause. Eating enough protein, avoiding sugar, consuming healthy fats, drinking green tea, eating a lot of fatty fish, learning to manage your stress, and getting as much sleep as possible.

Insomnia

Create a sleep-friendly environment. Turn off all electronic devices. Do not bring your phones, laptops, etc. into your bedroom. Turn that television off, better yet do not have one in the bedroom.

Eat at least two hours before bed. But if you do need a snack before bed, it should not be wine, chocolate, or anything that contains caffeine which is a stimulant.

Try to avoid drinking at least an hour before bed.

Try essential oils such as lavender.

Bedroom temperature, types of sheets, and mattress can all affect your sleep. Try for a quiet, dark, and cool environment.

Establish a sleep routine. A routine is very important to establishing good sleep. Take a calming bath or listen to some relaxing music.

Maintaining healthy relationships and being socially active with intellectual stimulation can help with your sleep.

Exercise studies show that regular exercise can improve sleep quality. Try 30 minutes of moderate-intensity activity during the day. Exercising too close to bedtime can be stimulating so watch the timing of your workout.

Healthy eating is essential, try foods that increase melatonin levels such as walnuts which cause the brain to secrete melatonin.

Almonds contain a sleep-enhancing amino acid called tryptophan. Almonds also contain magnesium which relaxes our muscles for a good night sleep.

Tryptophan is also found in cheese.

Lettuce contains a substance with sedative properties called lactucarium.

Tuna contains vitamin B6 which is needed to produce melatonin.

Try juicing some cherries which have both melatonin and tryptophan.

Chamomile tea contains properties that make it a mild tranquilizer and sleep inducer.

Use honey in your chamomile tea. Studies show that raw honey consumed during the day will promote restful sleep.

Fish such as salmon, tuna, and halibut has vitamin B6 which the body needs to produce melatonin. You can also get vitamin B6 from raw garlic and pistachios.

Kale, spinach, and mustard greens are high in calcium which the brain needs to create melatonin and tryptophan.

Ashwagandha is considered an adaptogen (an herb that protects the body). Research shows that it may help you to fall asleep faster, stay asleep longer, and have a better quality of sleep.

L-theanine is found in green tea, mushrooms; other kinds of teas such as some oolong, and some types of black tea. L-theanine is said to impact the neurotransmitters involved with sleep, stress, mood, and focus and enhances the production of serotonin and dopamine.

Magnesium is so very important. It plays a role in over 300 biochemical reactions in the body. It protects bones and teeth, helps to maintain normal muscle and nerve function, and it supports the reduction of tiredness and fatigue. It activates the parasympathetic nervous system which is responsible for promoting feelings of calmness and relaxation. Studies show that it encourages deep restorative sleep and improves sleep quality. It may help in combatting depression. Every woman should be taking magnesium.

CBD and 5HTP may also help with your sleep. Do your research and talk to professionals before taking any medicines or supplements.

RESERVE BED FOR SEX AND SLEEP (it is not your office)!

Anger

Anger is another real symptom of menopause. With everything going on as a result of the lack of hormones, it's typical that we should feel emotional and even angry. You are producing less estrogen and less serotonin so this will directly impact how stable and optimistic you will feel. Those hot flashes, vaginal dryness, lack of sleep, lack of sex, gaining weight, hair falling out, and so many more symptoms that you may have just suddenly begun to experience will have you frustrated and angry at times. However, this does not mean that you have permanently lost control over the way you feel.

Try eating a diet rich in vitamin D, calcium, and iron to balance your hormones.

Because we tend to gain weight during menopause try foods rich in high fiber which will keep your digestion regular. Plant estrogen that is found in soy can also help with your menopausal symptoms so try foods such as tofu, edamame, and soy milk. Maintaining your previous weight and appearance will have a good effect on your emotions.

Use mediation, yoga, stress management, and mindfulness. Do deep breathing.

Channel your anger into a productive outlet. Painting, writing, gardening, decorating, etc. Try journaling, put your feelings and thoughts on paper. This way you can reflect at a later date and do what it takes to make necessary changes.

Do not be afraid to see your medical professional if you find that your behavior is getting erratic. If you are experiencing panic attacks or your relationships are suffering because of your anger, you are not to blame, there is a very real chemical reaction at play.

Depression

Depression is very real during menopause. You wake up one day, and your life has changed. One day, you are fine, and the next, you wake up with a heat coming from inside your body that you have never experienced before, and you are scared because your mother did not tell you about it, your doctor did not tell you about it, your girlfriends are not talking about it so you feel lost, alone, and scared. This could very well lead you into a form of depression.

Hormone changes are a noticeably big deal. The key here is to balance your hormones. Eat the foods mentioned previously. Foods like turkey, chicken, sesame seeds, and bananas all have tryptophan, a building block of that feel-good chemical serotonin. Soybeans and flaxseeds are a great source of phytoestrogen and mimic estrogen in your body.

Take the vitamins and supplements mentioned as well. Vitamin D is so very important. Red clover is another type of phytoestrogen that has a similar chemical makeup of estrogen. Black cohosh as well. Dong Quai is female ginseng that has been effective in restoring hormone levels. Chasteberry plant boost estrogen and progesterone levels and Maca also boost estrogen levels.

Vitamin B6 and Vitamin B12

Dark chocolate

Reducing alcohol; reducing sugar

Exercise is important, it can stimulate endorphin hormones which will improve your mood. Yoga and walking are great exercises.

Look at your life and see what may be causing your depression

If your depression is serious, see a medical professional who may prescribe an antidepressant or other medications.

HRT is also a possibility for some women, see your health care professional.

Look into methods such as Australian Bush Remedies or Bach Rescue Remedies. We can get online and do our research so we no longer have to suffer in silence.

Mood Swings

It's important to have healthy relationships, not have a lot of stress in your life, not have an unhealthy living situation, and of course, exercise, eat healthily, and follow all the previous remedies mentioned.

Try Mindfulness, Yoga, and Reiki. Have a creative outlet, find a hobby. Nurture great friendships. Avoid alcohol and tranquilizers.

Don't focus on the loss of your childbearing years and other changes, instead, focus on things that you love about yourself, identify the negative thoughts, and change them. Focus on things that make you happy. The positive things that this stage of life will bring.

Try ginseng, it helps to improve mood and sleep.

St John's Wort may help to reduce anxiety, depression, and mood swings.

Maco Root reduces anxiety and stress, it alleviates cortisol levels.

Black Cohosh alleviates hormone imbalance.

If your mood swings continue or become severe, see your doctor!

Night Sweats

First thing is to try to find your triggers and stay away from them. Some triggers might be smoking, wearing tight restrictive clothes, using heavy comforters and blankets, drinking alcohol or caffeine, eating spicy foods, stress, and rooms that are too hot.

Dress in layers so you can easily remove clothing when you are too hot.

Wear loose light clothing.

Have a bedside fan.

Turn your thermostat down before bedtime.

Keep water beside your bed for sipping.

Deep calm breathing exercises.

Use cooling sprays and gels.

Use the natural supplements and foods mentioned above to help balance your hormones. Evening primrose oil works wonders for my girlfriend but may do nothing for you, everyone is different. Supplements such as vitamin E will help with other symptoms as well like vaginal dryness. You can find vitamin E in wheat germ oil, peanuts, avocados, red sweet peppers, and mangoes.

As with all the other symptoms, you will need to get your hormones balanced. Eating right, exercising, trying to stay away from stress, and getting your supplements will all help you to have a better menopause experience.

Raw unfiltered apple cider vinegar may reduce perspiration and reduce the intensity of hot flashes and night sweats.

Incontinence

Dealing with incontinence can be both stressful and embarrassing. Bladder leakage when you cough, and when you exercise, and waking up often to pee during the night. However, there are small changes that you can make to help you regain control of your bladder. Use Kegel exercises to strengthen your pelvic muscles. These exercises will lower your risk of bowel and bladder issues and will also help to lower the risk of vaginal prolapse. Do pelvic floor exercises, you may want to visit a pelvic floor specialist if you are having these issues.

Avoid drinks with caffeine. Caffeine can cause the bladder and parts of the pelvic to become overactive because it is a diuretic and bladder irritant. It may cause inflammation of your bladder which will increase your urge to go to the bathroom.

Use vitamin D. Vitamin D affects skeletal muscle, strength, and function so insufficient vitamin D will affect bladder muscles as well.

Avoid alcohol, it can also act as a diuretic which may result in not only more urine production but also the need to go more frequently.

Smoking may cause an inflammation of the bladder. If you are experiencing incontinence, try to quit smoking.

Keep a log. Know how often you pee, how much you drink, each time you have an urge to pee, and how strong your urge is.

Bone Loss

To help you with bone loss, it's simply getting enough calcium and vitamin D. Have you noticed how vitamin D is mentioned everywhere? It is so necessary to the body and is more of a hormone instead of a vitamin. These are the two most important nutrients for bone health.

Calcium is necessary for life. It keeps our heart beating, builds bones, enables our blood to clot, and our muscles to contract. Every day, we lose calcium through our skin, feces, urine, hair, sweat, and nails. And because our bodies cannot produce calcium, we have to make sure we are replacing what we are losing. It's okay for our bodies to take some calcium from our bone once in a while, but the more it takes, the more our bones get weak and is easier to break.

It is recommended that women in their menopausal years take 1200 - 1500mg of calcium daily.

Foods rich in calcium are;

- Milk
- Cheeses
- Yogurt
- Turnip greens
- Collard greens
- Kale
- Bok Choy
- Oranges
- Sardines

- Almond milk, rice milk, and soy milk
- Beans

Vitamin D protects your bones by helping your body to absorb calcium. It is the support your muscles needed to avoid falls. Adults need vitamin D to keep their bones strong and healthy. It is recommended that women over the age of 50 take 800-1000IU daily. There are 3 ways to get your vitamin D, the sun, food, and supplements.

Your skin will make vitamin D when in the sun and store it in fat for use later on. The amount of vitamin D that your skin will produce depends on your pigmentation, the time of day, age, and season.

Vitamin D is also not found in a lot of food, so getting out in the sun is important.

You will need the vitamin D to absorb calcium, but you do not have to take both at the same time.

Estrogen

Estrogen is one of the major hormones in a woman's body, we have already discussed how estrogen production declines during perimenopause. However, there are natural ways of boosting your estrogen.

Foods such as:

- Flaxseed
- Soybeans
- Sesame seeds

- Cashews
- Pine nuts
- Sunflower seeds
- Pumpkin seeds
- Walnuts and Almond
- Peas and Garlic
- Vitamins and minerals such as Vitamin D and Vitamin B
- Baron
- DHEA
- Black Cohosh
- Chasteberry
- Red clover

As always, consult with your doctor or health care provider before using any of these supplements.

Progesterone

Progesterone, in combination with estrogen, will help to alleviate some of your perimenopause symptoms. Foods do not necessarily contain progesterone, but some foods which are believed to stimulate the body's production of progesterone are:

- Beans
- Broccoli
- Brussels sprouts

- Cabbage
- Cauliflower
- Kale
- Nuts
- Pumpkin seeds
- Spinach
- Whole grains
- Dark chocolate
- Citrus
- Leafy greens
- Peppers
- Salmon
- Shrimp
- Oats
- Cruciferous vegetables

Foods to Avoid

There are certain types of foods that you should avoid during menopause. These foods could act as triggers and make your symptoms worsen.

Spicy foods will trigger sweating, flushing, and hot flashes.

Processed foods have added sugar and are generally high in sodium. And because sugar is easily digested and enters the bloodstream quickly it makes the blood glucose level high. This in turn will worsen your menopause symptoms. Studies have shown that women with higher blood sugar levels have more frequent hot flashes, regardless of their estrogen levels. This can also promote heart disease and weight gain.

Fast foods and fried foods are also foods to avoid. Studies have shown that eating fried foods contributes to an increase in heart-related deaths in post-menopausal women.

Foods that are high in carbs such as pasta, potatoes, white loaves of bread, and rice may also contribute to fatigue and moodiness.

Water

Water is always important to the human body, but during menopause, we lose estrogen which helps to keep us hydrated, this means that we lose the ability to retain water. So, during menopause, you have to make sure you are drinking enough water to keep your body hydrated. Also remember that with numerous hot flashes and sweating during the day and night, you are constantly losing water so you will need to make sure you are constantly hydrating.

Drinking 8-10 glasses of water a day can help with your menopause symptoms and helps to reduce bloating. Drinking 500ml of water before dinner may help you to consume fewer calories during your meal and that will help with weight gain/loss.

Water is important for:

- Joints—dehydration can cause inflammation.

- Skin—dehydration can cause itchy skin and causes your skin to look rough and wrinkled.

- Mood—dehydration can cause mood swings, anxiety, and panic attacks.

- Memory—dehydration can cause brain fog, fuzziness, and forgetfulness.

- Headaches—dehydration is a trigger for headaches.

- Constipation/bloating—dehydration slows down your gut motility and elimination of feces.

- Fatigue—dehydration can affect energy levels.

- Hot flashes—can affect the nervous system which triggers hot flashes.

Note; fancy waters, fizzy water, and flavored water do not count as your daily water intake.

Exercise

According to the center for disease control and prevention, most healthy women should be getting 150 minutes of moderate aerobic activity or 75 minutes of vigorous aerobic activity per week. Start with 10 minutes per day and slowly increase as it gets easier.

Walking, jogging, biking, and swimming are all great ways to use your large muscle groups while keeping up your heart rate. Start with 10 minutes. Strength training is important during menopause because we lose bone. Strength training exercises will build bone and muscle strength. It will burn body fat and help with your metabolism.

Yoga can be greatly beneficial during menopause. Restorative yoga requires that your poses are held longer, often with the support of a prop such as a folded blanket. Supportive and restorative yoga may help to calm your nerves by centering your mind and relaxing the nervous system and to alleviate such symptoms like hot flashes, fatigue, irritability, stress, depression, and mood swings.

HRT Hormone Replace Therapy

Hormone replacement therapy replenishes the hormones that are diminished during menopause. This will help to relieve the symptoms of menopause. Speak to your doctor who can explain the different types of replacement therapy and help you to get on the correct dosage for you.

HRT may not be suitable for some women. Women who have a history of breast cancer, ovarian cancer, womb cancer, history of blood clots, untreated high blood pressure, and liver disease should not have HRT.

Self-care

Take the time for yourself, for personal things, and hobbies. Self-care is learning to say "no" and putting yourself first. Women tend to help everyone around them and put themselves last, neglecting their own needs. Menopause is a time for you to focus on your own needs, finally putting yourself first. Speak up for yourself, it is okay to need time for yourself, and it's ok to not show up for everyone who needs you; you need you. You don't have to feel guilty, you have done so much, and it's your time now. Do what you have to do for yourself, be gentle to yourself!

SUMMARY

It is so important to be at our healthiest during menopause. Not only will being in optimal health help lessen our symptoms, but it will also decrease your risk of diseases such as heart disease and osteoporosis.

Managing your symptoms will also have a better effect on your overall life. During menopause, communication can become strained between partners which can lead to a relationship issue. Over 60% of divorces are initiated by women in their menopausal years. And over $150 billion in productivity is lost per year due to menopause. Women are leaving their relationships and careers. A lot of us do not know where to begin and what questions to start asking. We are ashamed to talk about our symptoms or we do not even know that what we are experiencing are symptoms of menopause.

I hope this will explain a few things and get you started on your journey to a better menopausal life. This is just the ABCs to get you started so you can now start asking about the DEFs and so forth.

I wish you an easy and safe menopausal journey!

REFERENCES

https://www.everydayhealth.com

American menopause society

https://www.yogajournal.com

https://askthescientists.com

https://www.healthline.com

https://www.health.harvard.edu

https://www.bonehealthandosteoporosis.org

https://www.womens-health-concern.org

https://www.medicalnewstoday.com

www.ingramcontent.com/pod-product-compliance
Lightning Source LLC
Chambersburg PA
CBHW071126030426
42336CB00013BA/2224